FITNESS AT HOME
Building a Home Gym and Crafting an Effective Workout Routine
By
Anjela Smith

Dedication:
This Book is dedicated to all individuals who are committed to improving their fitness and overall well-being from the comfort of their own homes.

Table Of Contents

INTRODUCTION

In today's fast-paced world, finding time to prioritize our health and fitness can often be a challenge. However, there is a growing trend that is revolutionizing the way we approach exercise – home workouts. More and more people are discovering the convenience and effectiveness of building a home gym and crafting an effective workout routine in the comfort of their own space.

The growing trend of home workouts and the benefits of exercising at home:

With busy schedules and limited access to gyms, many individuals are turning to the idea of exercising at home. This trend has been fueled by advancements in technology, the availability of home workout equipment, and the desire for a more flexible and convenient fitness routine. Working out at home allows you to say goodbye to crowded gyms, long commutes, and strict gym hours. Not only does exercising at home save time, but it also offers a multitude of benefits for your overall well-being. When you exercise at home, you have complete control over your workout environment – from the music you enjoy, to the temperature, and even the company you keep. Additionally, home workouts provide a level of privacy and comfort that can enhance your exercise experience.

Overview of the book's purpose and what readers will gain from it: In "Fitness at Home: Building a Home Gym and Crafting an Effective Workout Routine," our aim is to guide you on your journey to building a home gym and creating a workout routine that works for you. With comprehensive strategies and expert advice, this book will equip you with the knowledge and resources needed to transform your home into a fitness sanctuary.

Throughout the chapters, we will delve into various aspects of home workouts, including setting up your home gym, designing an effective workout routine, incorporating cardio and strength training, improving flexibility and mobility, and overcoming challenges to stay motivated. We will also explore advanced home workouts, maintenance and safety tips, and strategies for staying active while traveling.

By the end of this book, you will have gained a thorough understanding of the advantages of exercising at home and the tools necessary to succeed in your fitness journey. Whether you are a beginner or an experienced fitness enthusiast, "Fitness at Home" will serve as your invaluable resource for creating a home gym that suits your needs, and crafting a workout routine that will help you achieve your health and fitness goals. Get ready to unlock your full potential and embark on a rewarding journey to a healthier and fitter you from the comfort of your own home.

CHAPTER ONE

Setting Up Your Home Gym

Assessing Available Space and Budget Considerations

Before diving into setting up your home gym, it's important to assess the available space in your home and consider your budget. These factors will help determine what type of equipment and layout will work best for you. Here are a few things to keep in mind:

Space: Take a good look at the area you have designated for your home gym. Measure the dimensions of the space, ensuring you have enough room for the equipment you plan to include. Consider factors like ceiling height, ventilation, and accessibility.

Budget: Determine your budget for setting up your home gym. This will help you make informed decisions about the equipment you can afford and prioritize which pieces are essential.

Multi-Purpose Space: If you have limited space or a tight budget, consider selecting equipment that can be easily folded, stackable, or stored away when not in use. This allows you to use your gym space for other activities as well.

Necessary Equipment for a Basic Home Gym Setup

Setting up a home gym doesn't require a massive collection of equipment. You can achieve a great workout with just a few key pieces. Consider including the following items in your basic home gym setup:

Exercise Mat: An exercise mat provides a comfortable and non-slip surface for a variety
of exercises, such as stretching, yoga, and bodyweight exercises.

Dumbbells: Dumbbells are versatile and can be used for various strength training exercises. Start with a few different weights that suit your current fitness level and gradually increase as you progress.

Resistance Bands: Resistance bands are affordable, lightweight, and portable. They can be used for strength training, stretching, and rehabilitation exercises.

Jump Rope: Jumping rope is an excellent cardiovascular exercise that can be done in a small space. It offers a high-intensity workout and helps improve coordination and endurance.

Stability Ball: Stability balls are great for core strengthening exercises, balance training, and improving posture. They come in various sizes, so choose one that suits your height.

Tips for Organizing and Optimizing Your Workout Space

To create a functional and enjoyable workout space, consider the following tips for organizing and optimizing your home gym:

Clear the Space: Remove any unnecessary clutter or furniture from the designated workout area. This will create a clear space for your exercise routine and reduce the risk of accidents or distractions.

Proper Lighting: Ensure that the area has adequate lighting, either natural or artificial. Good lighting helps you focus on your exercises and minimizes the risk of injuries.

Flooring: Choose a suitable flooring option for your home gym. Opt for materials that provide cushioning and reduce impact, such as foam tiles or rubber flooring.

Equipment Placement: Place your equipment strategically to maximize space and facilitate a smooth workout flow. Consider wall-mounted storage racks or shelves to keep your equipment organized and easily accessible.

Mirrors: Installing mirrors on one or more walls can help you monitor your form during exercises. Mirrors also create an illusion of a larger space and enhance the overall aesthetic appeal.

Ventilation and Climate Control: Ensure proper ventilation and temperature control in your home gym to keep the air fresh and comfortable during workouts. A fan or air purifier can be beneficial.

Remember, your home gym setup should be tailored to your individual needs and preferences. Consider your fitness goals, available space, and budget when selecting equipment and organizing your workout area. With a well-thought-out setup, you'll have a functional and motivating home gym that sets the stage for a successful fitness journey

CHAPTER TWO

Cardiovascular Fitness

Understanding the Importance of Cardio Workouts for Overall Fitness

In this chapter, we will delve into the significance of cardiovascular fitness for achieving overall fitness and maintaining a healthy lifestyle. Cardio workouts offer tremendous benefits that extend beyond weight loss. Regular cardiovascular exercise improves heart health, increases lung capacity, reduces the risk of chronic diseases, enhances mood, boosts energy levels, and promotes better sleep.

By engaging in cardio exercises, you can improve your cardiovascular endurance, which refers to the ability of your heart and lungs to supply oxygen and blood to your working muscles efficiently. This, in turn, allows you to engage in a wide range of physical activities with ease and less fatigue. Understanding the pivotal role that cardiovascular fitness plays in your overall well-being will motivate you to incorporate cardio workouts into your home gym routine.

Exploring Various Cardio Exercises Suitable for Home Workouts

Now that we comprehend the significance of cardiovascular fitness, it's time to explore a variety of cardio exercises that are suitable for home workouts. The beauty of performing cardio exercises at home is the flexibility to choose activities that align with your preferences and available space.

Jumping Jacks: A classic exercise that requires minimal space, jumping jacks effectively elevate your heart rate and engage multiple muscle groups. You can easily modify the intensity by increasing the speed and incorporating variations like cross jacks or star jumps.

High Knees: This exercise involves marching or jogging in place while lifting your knees as high as possible. High knees effectively target your lower body while increasing your heart rate, making it an excellent cardio exercise that can be performed in small spaces.

Skipping Rope: A cost-effective home workout tool, a skipping rope is perfect for cardiovascular exercise. Skipping rope improves coordination, agility, and cardiovascular endurance. With a variety of techniques like double under or alternating foot skips, this exercise can be adapted to different fitness levels.

Kickboxing: Incorporating kickboxing moves into your routine provides an intense cardiovascular workout while also working on your coordination, flexibility, and strength. Online kickboxing tutorials or DVDs can guide you on performing proper techniques for an effective home workout.

Strategies for Maximizing Cardio Gains at Home

To maximize your cardio gains when working out at home, it's important to employ effective strategies that challenge your cardiovascular fitness and ensure progression. Consider the following tips:

Set Measurable Goals: Establish specific and realistic goals, such as increasing your workout duration or intensity week by week. By tracking your progress, you'll stay motivated and experience continual improvements in your cardiovascular fitness.

Interval Training: Incorporate interval training into your cardio workouts by alternating between periods of high-intensity exercises and recovery periods. This technique not only enhances your cardiovascular endurance but also increases calorie burning and metabolic rate.

Mix Up Your Workouts: Avoid monotony and boredom by incorporating a variety of cardio exercises into your routine. Experiment with different activities such as dancing, stair climbing, or cycling to challenge your body and keep your workouts exciting.

Monitor Your Heart Rate: Invest in a heart rate monitor or utilize smartphone apps that can track your heart rate during workouts. This will allow you to ensure you're hitting the desired intensity levels and tailor your workouts to suit your fitness goals.

By implementing these strategies, you can effectively maximize your cardiovascular gains, make progress, and gradually achieve your desired fitness level.

Remember, the journey to cardiovascular fitness starts from the comfort of your own home. With the right understanding, suitable exercises, and smart strategies, you can transform your home gym into a powerhouse for enhancing your overall fitness through cardiovascular workouts. In the next chapter, we will shift our focus to resistance training and building strength at home.

CHAPTER THREE

Strength Training

Welcome to Chapter 3 of "Fitness at Home: Building a Home Gym and Crafting an Effective Workout Routine." In this chapter, we will focus on the significance of strength training and building muscle at home. We will also discuss the various types of strength training equipment suitable for a home gym and provide guidelines for designing a balanced strength training routine incorporating bodyweight exercises and equipment.

Section A:
The Benefits of Strength Training and Building Muscle at Home

Strength training plays a vital role in improving overall fitness and achieving optimal health. Here are some key benefits of strength training and building muscle at home:
Increased Muscle Mass: Regular strength training exercises stimulate muscle growth, leading to increased muscle mass and strength. This not only enhances your physical appearance but also improves your ability to perform daily tasks efficiently.
Improved Bone Density: Strength training is crucial for maintaining and increasing bone density, especially as we age. It helps to prevent conditions such as osteoporosis and reduces the risk of fractures. By engaging in strength training at home, you can strengthen your skeletal system and promote long-term bone health.
Enhanced Metabolism: Strength training supports weight loss and weight management by boosting your metabolism. As you build lean muscle mass, your body utilizes calories more efficiently, even at rest. This increased metabolic rate aids in burning fat and achieving a leaner physique.
Increased Functional Strength: Daily activities like lifting, carrying groceries, or playing with children require strength and endurance. Strength training at home improves functional strength, enabling you to perform these tasks with greater ease and reducing the risk of injuries.
Improved Mental Health: Engaging in strength training not only benefits your physical health but also improves your mental well-being. Regular workouts release endorphins, the feel-good

hormones, reducing stress, anxiety, and symptoms of depression.

Section B:

Overview of Different Types of Strength Training Equipment for a Home Gym

When considering strength training at home, it's essential to select suitable equipment that fits your needs and space constraints. Here's an overview of different types of strength training equipment ideal for a home gym:

Dumbbells: Versatile and effective, dumbbells are a must-have for any home gym. They come in various weights and can be used for a wide range of exercises, targeting different muscle groups.

Resistance Bands: An excellent choice for those starting with strength training or looking for portable equipment. Resistance bands offer various resistance levels and can be easily incorporated into bodyweight exercises to add intensity.

Barbell and Weight Plates: If you have space and are looking to perform compound lifts like squats, deadlifts, and bench presses, investing in a barbell and weight plates is a great option. This combination allows for progressive overload and is suitable for advanced lifters.

Suspension Trainer: These versatile systems use straps to leverage body weight, offering a full-body workout. Suspension trainers are compact and easy to set up, making them an excellent addition to any home gym.

Section C:

Designing a Balanced Strength Training Routine Using Bodyweight Exercises and Equipment

To create an effective and balanced strength training routine at home, consider incorporating both bodyweight exercises and equipment. Here are some guidelines to help you design your workout routine:

Start with Bodyweight Exercises: Begin your routine with bodyweight exercises such as push-ups, squats, lunges, planks, and burgees. These exercises engage multiple muscle groups simultaneously and serve as an excellent foundation for strength training.

Progress to Equipment-Based Exercises: As you gain strength and confidence, start incorporating equipment-based exercises. Utilize dumbbells, resistance bands, or barbells to add resistance and create more challenging workouts.

Follow a Split Routine: Divide your training sessions to focus on specific muscle groups on different days. For example, you can have a day dedicated to upper body exercises, another for lower body exercises, and a third day for core and full-body workouts.

Aim for Progressive Overload: To continually challenge your muscles and promote muscle growth, gradually increase the resistance or intensity of your exercises. This can be achieved by adding more weight, increasing repetitions, or reducing rest times.

Conclusion:

Incorporating strength training into your fitness routine at home offers numerous benefits for your physical and mental well-being. By understanding the benefits of strength training, selecting appropriate equipment, and designing a balanced workout routine, you are well on your way to achieving your fitness goals. In Chapter 5, we will explore the importance of cardiovascular exercise and how to incorporate it effectively into your home gym workouts. Stay motivated and keep striving for a healthier and fitter you!

CHAPTER FOUR

Flexibility

and Mobility

In the previous chapters, we have discussed the importance of setting up a home gym and crafting an effective workout routine. However, no fitness regimen is complete without addressing a vital aspect – flexibility and mobility. This chapter will shed light on the significance of flexibility and mobility exercises in preventing injuries, explore various stretching and mobility routines suitable for home workouts, and demonstrate how to incorporate tools like foam rollers and resistance bands to enhance flexibility.

By focusing on these three items, you'll unlock the immense benefits of a well-rounded fitness routine that not only builds strength but also ensures overall injury prevention and improved performance.

A. Importance of flexibility and mobility exercises in preventing injuries:

1. Understanding the anatomy behind injuries:

   a. The role of muscle imbalances and posture in injury susceptibility.

   b. How limited mobility can increase the risk of sprains, strains, and tears.

   c. The relationship between flexibility, mobility, and overall joint health.

2. The benefits of regular flexibility and mobility training:

   a. Improved range of motion and joint stability.

   b. Enhancing muscle performance and avoiding overcompensation.

   c. Reducing the likelihood of chronic pain and promoting proper alignment.

   d. Enhancing overall athletic and functional abilities.

3. Addressing misconceptions about flexibility:

   a. Debunking the notion that stretching is only for athletes.

   b. Highlighting the advantages of incorporating flexibility exercises in any fitness routine.

   c. The correlation between improved flexibility and better posture.

B. Exploring different stretching and mobility routines for home workouts:

1. Dynamic stretching:

a. Understanding dynamic stretching and its contribution to workout performance.

b. Demonstrating dynamic warm-up routines for different muscle groups.

2. Static stretching:

a. Explaining the benefits and correct techniques of static stretching.

b. Presenting a comprehensive full-body static stretching routine for post-workout relaxation and injury prevention.

3. Active isolated stretching:

a. Introducing the concept of active isolated stretching and its role in rehabilitation and functional mobility.

b. Demonstrating simple active isolated stretching exercises tailored for home workouts.

C. Incorporating tools such as foam rollers and resistance bands for improved flexibility:

1. The benefits of foam rolling:

a. Explaining myofascial release and its positive effects on muscle recovery and flexibility.

b. Demonstrating foam roller exercises targeting major muscle groups.

2. Harnessing the power of resistance bands:

a. Outlining the versatility and advantages of resistance band training.

b. Presenting a range of resistance band exercises to enhance flexibility and mobility.

Conclusion:

Flexibility and mobility exercises are often overlooked aspects of a fitness routine. However, by dedicating time and effort to improve these areas, you can safeguard yourself from injuries, boost your performance, and achieve optimal results. In this chapter, we discussed the importance of flexibility and mobility exercises in injury prevention, explored various stretching and mobility routines suitable for home workouts, and highlighted the benefits of incorporating tools like foam rollers and resistance bands to enhance flexibility. By prioritizing flexibility and mobility, you are investing in long-term physical well-being and unlocking your body's limitless potential.

CHAPTER FIVE

Creating an Effective

Workout Routine

Congratulations on reaching Chapter 5 of "Fitness at Home: Building a Home Gym and Crafting an Effective Workout Routine." In this chapter, we will delve into the crucial aspects of creating an effective workout routine that aligns with your personal goals, available time, and prevents plateaus. By implementing the strategies discussed in this chapter, you will be well on your way to achieving your desired level of fitness and surpassing your own expectations.

A. Goal-setting and Determining Individual Fitness Objectives
Before embarking on any workout routine, it is essential to establish your

goals and understand your individual fitness objectives. This introspective process will help you stay motivated and focused throughout your fitness journey. Begin by asking yourself what you hope to achieve through your workouts. Is it weight loss, muscle gain, improved flexibility, or increased stamina? Be specific in defining your goals, and consider setting both short-term and long-term objectives.

Once you have identified your fitness objectives, it's important to assess your current fitness level and any limitations you may have. Consult with a healthcare professional if necessary and keep in mind that everyone's fitness journey is unique. By setting realistic and attainable goals, you can celebrate small victories along the way, further fueling your motivation.

B.Designing a Workout Routine that Aligns with Personal Goals and Available Time

Designing a workout routine that aligns with your personal goals and fits into your schedule is vital for long-term adherence. Consider the following factors when crafting your routine:

Frequency: Determine how many days per week you can realistically commit to exercising. Strive for a balance between consistency and giving your body adequate time to rest and recover.

Time: Assess your daily routine and identify windows of time that you can consistently dedicate to working out. Whether it's in the morning, during your lunch break, or in the evening, choose a time that allows you to focus and enjoy your workouts without feeling rushed.

Workout Types: Select exercises and training methods that align with your individual goals. For example, if muscle gain is your primary goal, focus on resistance training exercises. If weight loss is your focus, incorporate a combination of cardio and strength training.

Variety: Incorporate a variety of exercises and workout styles to keep your routine engaging and prevent boredom. This can include bodyweight exercises, weightlifting, cardio intervals, yoga, or any other activity you enjoy.

By designing a workout routine tailored to your goals and availability, you will be more likely to stick with it in the long run.

Structuring Workouts for Optimal Effectiveness and Preventing Plateaus

To ensure optimal effectiveness and ongoing progress, it is crucial to structure your workouts strategically:

Warm-up: Begin each session with a dynamic warm-up to prepare your muscles and joints for the upcoming exercises. Incorporate movements that mimic the exercises you will be performing.

Main Workout: Structure your workouts to target different muscle groups or fitness components on different days. This approach allows for adequate recovery and minimizes the risk of overtraining. Consider incorporating compound exercises that work multiple muscle groups simultaneously for efficiency.

Progression: Gradually increase the intensity, duration, or resistance of your workouts as you become more comfortable with the exercises. Progression is key to prevent plateaus and continually challenge your body. Recovery: Integrate rest days into your weekly routine to allow your body to recover and adapt. Overtraining can lead to fatigue, injury, and hinder progress. Listen to your body and adjust your routine accordingly. Remember, consistency and dedication are essential when it comes to achieving your fitness goals. By following these guidelines, you will create a workout routine that is not only effective but also enjoyable and sustainable over the long term.
In the next chapter, we will explore nutrition and its role in fueling your workouts and optimizing your overall fitness.

CHAPTER SIX

Overcoming Challenges

and Staying Motivated

In order to achieve your fitness goals, it is essential to address the common barriers that may hinder your progress when working out at home. This chapter will provide you with practical strategies to overcome these obstacles, as well as tips for staying motivated and accountable to your fitness routine. Additionally, incorporating variety and tracking progress will ensure continued enthusiasm on your fitness journey.

A. Addressing Common Barriers to Exercising at Home and Strategies to Overcome Them

1. Lack of equipment: Many individuals assume they cannot effectively exercise at home due to a perceived need for expensive gym equipment. However, there are numerous ways to exercise using minimal or no equipment. This section will explore bodyweight exercises, household items as workout tools, and budget-friendly equipment alternatives.

2. Limited space: Another common challenge in setting up a home gym is the misconception that a large space is necessary. This section will highlight creative ways to utilize small spaces efficiently, such as utilizing walls, corners, or even clearing furniture temporarily for workout sessions. Additionally, it will discuss the benefits of outdoor workouts or modifying exercises to suit the available space.

3. Distractions and lack of privacy: Finding focus and creating a dedicated workout space can be difficult when exercising at home. This section will provide strategies to minimize distractions, including setting boundaries with family members or roommates, establishing a workout schedule, and creating a designated workout area. Additionally, it will explore using headphones, white noise machines, or motivational playlists to increase concentration.

B. Tips for Staying Motivated and Accountable to Your Fitness Routine

1. Set realistic goals: Establishing achievable fitness goals is crucial for maintaining motivation. This section will guide you on setting SMART (Specific, Measurable, Attainable, Relevant, Time-bound) goals and breaking them down into smaller milestones. It will also emphasize the importance of celebrating progress along the way.

2. Find a workout buddy or support system: Exercising with a partner or joining online fitness communities can significantly boost motivation and accountability. This section will explore the benefits of finding a workout buddy, whether in-person or virtually, and how to create a supportive network that keeps you on track.

3. Track progress and celebrate achievements: Incorporating progress tracking methods, such as fitness journals or mobile apps, will help you visualize your progress and motivate you to keep going. This section will discuss various ways to track your workouts, measure improvements, and reward yourself for achieving milestones.

C. Incorporating Variety and Tracking Progress for Continued Enthusiasm

1. Spice up your fitness routine: Repetitive workouts can lead to boredom and decreased motivation. This section will provide ideas for incorporating variety into your home fitness routine, such as trying different

workout styles, exploring online
workout classes, or experimenting
with new equipment or exercises.
2. Set regular challenges or
milestones: Introducing challenges or
milestones can inject excitement into
your fitness journey. Whether it's
participating in a virtual race,
completing a 30-day fitness challenge,
or conquering a new exercise, these
goals will help maintain enthusiasm
and drive. This section will explore
various challenges and milestones
that can be integrated into your
routine.
3. Reflect and adjust: Regularly
evaluating your progress and
adjusting your workout routine
accordingly is vital for sustained
motivation. This section will guide you
on reviewing your fitness journey,
identifying areas of improvement, and
adjusting your routine to avoid
plateaus or boredom.
Conclusion: Overcoming challenges
and staying motivated throughout your
fitness journey is essential to
achieving long-term success. By
addressing common barriers, staying
accountable, and incorporating variety
while tracking progress, you will
ensure continued enthusiasm and
reap the benefits of working out at
home.

CHAPTER SEVEN

Advanced

Home Workouts

Progressing beyond basic workouts and adding complexity to routines Congratulations! If you've reached Chapter Seven, it means you've successfully mastered the basics of home workouts. Now, it's time to take your fitness journey to the next level by progressing beyond the basic workouts and adding complexity to your routines. This chapter will guide you on how to make your workouts more challenging, effective, and enjoyable.

Understanding progressive overload: To continue seeing progress, it's essential to challenge your body by progressively increasing the intensity, duration, or frequency of your workouts. Learn how to incrementally overload your muscles, cardiovascular system, and flexibility to promote continuous improvement.

Incorporating circuit and interval training: Circuit and interval training are excellent ways to add complexity to your routines. They involve performing a combination of exercises in a specific order with minimal rest. Discover different circuit and interval training formats that suit your fitness goals and learn how to structure and design your own challenging workouts.

Utilizing advanced training techniques: Explore various advanced training techniques such as supersets, drop sets, pyramid sets, and partial reps. These techniques help increase muscle strength, size, and endurance by pushing your body beyond its limits. Learn how to incorporate these techniques into your routines effectively and safely.

Incorporating advanced exercises and techniques for continued challenge

Once you've mastered the basics, it's time to introduce advanced exercises and techniques into your home workout routine. These exercises and techniques will provide you with new challenges, break plateaus, and keep your sessions exciting. In this section, we'll explore some popular advanced exercises and techniques.

Plyometric exercises: Plyometric involve explosive movements that promote power, speed, and agility. Learn how to perform exercises like box jumps, burgees, and split squat jumps to enhance your performance, burn more calories, and improve overall body strength.

Advanced bodyweight exercises: Push-ups, squats, and lunges are great foundational exercises, but you can take them to the next level. Discover variations like one-arm push-ups, pistol squats, and Bulgarian split squats that target different muscle groups and challenge your balance and stability.

Incorporating resistance bands and weights: If you want to increase the intensity of your workouts, incorporating resistance bands and weights is the way to go. Learn how to properly utilize equipment like resistance bands, dumbbells, or kettlebells to enhance your strength and develop a more muscular physique.

Tips for maintaining safety and injury prevention during advanced home workouts

As you embark on more challenging workouts, it becomes even more crucial to prioritize safety and injury prevention. Follow these tips to minimize the risk of injuries during your advanced home workouts.

Warm-up and cool-down: Before diving into your intense workout, always begin with a dynamic warm-up routine to prepare your body for the upcoming challenges. Similarly, once you finish your workout, perform a proper cool-down, including static stretches, to improve flexibility and aid in muscle recovery.

Focus on proper form and technique: As you add complexity and intensity to your routines, it's essential to maintain proper form and technique. Poor form not only leads to inefficient workouts but also increases the risk of injury. If you're unsure about proper execution, seek guidance from fitness professionals or watch instructional videos to ensure you're performing exercises correctly.

Listen to your body: Advanced workouts push your limits, but it's crucial to listen to your body's signals. If you experience excessive pain, fatigue, or dizziness, take a break or modify your exercises accordingly.

Pushing through pain may lead to severe injuries or setbacks, so be mindful of your body's limitations.

In Conclusion

By progressing beyond basic workouts, incorporating advanced exercises and techniques, and prioritizing safety, you are on your way to achieving remarkable fitness goals from the comfort of your own home. Remember, consistency, dedication, and continued learning are the keys to success in your fitness at-home journey. Keep pushing your limits, and enjoy the incredible results these advanced home workouts will bring.

CHAPTER EIGHT

Maintaining Equipment and Safety

In this chapter, we will delve into the crucial aspects of maintaining your home gym equipment to ensure its longevity and functionality. Additionally, we will discuss the significance of creating a safe workout environment at home and outline common safety considerations and precautions during your home workouts. By implementing these practices, you will not only safeguard yourself from potential injuries but also maximize the effectiveness of your fitness routine.

Section A: Proper maintenance and care of home gym equipment

1. Regular Equipment Inspection:

   a. Emphasize the importance of regularly inspecting your home gym equipment for any signs of wear and tear or malfunction.

   b. Provide a checklist of key components to assess, such as cables, frames, handles, and padding.

   c. Offer tips for addressing minor repairs and maintenance, such as lubricating moving parts and tightening loose bolts.

2. Cleaning and Sanitizing:

   a. Discuss the significance of maintaining cleanliness in your home gym.

   b. Provide guidance on proper cleaning techniques for different types of equipment, including weights, mats, cardio machines, and benches.

   c. Highlight the benefits of sanitizing equipment regularly to minimize the transmission of germs and bacteria.

3. Storing Equipment:

   a. Offer tips on proper equipment storage to prevent damage and ensure safety.

   b. Discuss space-saving solutions for small home gyms.

   c. Explain how to store equipment properly, taking weight distribution and potential hazards into consideration.

Section B: Ensuring a safe workout environment at home

1. Adequate Space and Flooring:

   a. Highlight the importance of having sufficient space for safe and effective workouts.

   b. Provide recommendations for flooring options that offer appropriate cushioning and non-slip surfaces.

   c. Discuss the potential hazards of using equipment in confined areas or on unsuitable surfaces.

2. Proper Ventilation and Lighting:

a. Explain the significance of good ventilation to ensure the air quality in your home gym.

b. Discuss the importance of adequate lighting to prevent accidents and maintain visibility during workouts.

c. Offer suggestions for optimizing ventilation and lighting in your home gym setup.

3. Emergency Access and Communication:

a. Emphasize the necessity of easy access to emergency exits and phone communication during workouts.

b. Provide guidelines on ensuring that emergency contact information is readily available.

c. Discuss the importance of having a reliable means of communication within your home gym, such as a landline or cellphone.

Section C: Common safety considerations and precautions during home workouts

1. Warming up and Cooling Down:

a. Explain the significance of incorporating proper warm-up and cool-down routines.

b. Provide a step-by-step guide for an effective warm-up and cool-down session.

c. Highlight the benefits of warming up, including injury prevention and improved performance.

2. Proper Form and Technique:

a. Stress the importance of maintaining proper form and technique during exercises.

b. Provide visual references or links to resources demonstrating correct execution of common exercises.

c. Offer tips for self-assessing and correcting form errors to prevent injuries and optimize results.
3. Progression and Gradual Intensity:
a. Explain the concept of gradual progression and avoiding abrupt increases in workout intensity.
b. Provide guidance on incorporating progressive overload safely into your fitness routine.
c. Emphasize the importance of listening to your body's signals and adjusting intensity levels accordingly.
Conclusion:
By giving due attention to proper maintenance and care of your home gym equipment, ensuring a safe workout environment, and following common safety considerations and precautions, you will create an ideal setting for achieving fitness goals while minimizing the risk of injuries. Remember, safety should always be a priority to foster a long-term and enjoyable fitness journey at home.

CHAPTER NINE

Taking Your Home Gym

on the Go

Maintaining a fitness routine is essential, even when traveling. Whether you're on a business trip or enjoying a vacation, it's important to stay active and prioritize your health. In this chapter, we will explore strategies for staying active and maintaining fitness while traveling, portable equipment and workout routines for workouts on the go, as well as utilizing technology and online resources for home workouts away from home.

Strategies to" Staying Active and Maintaining Fitness while Traveling:

1. Plan Ahead:

   a. Research the available fitness facilities or gyms at your travel destination.

   b. Pack appropriate workout attire and shoes to ensure you're prepared for exercise.

2. Bodyweight Exercises:

   a. Explore bodyweight exercises that require no equipment, such as push-ups, squats, lunges, and planks.

   b. Create a short circuit workout routine that targets different muscle groups and can be done in a small space, like your hotel room.

3. Incorporate Physical Activities:

   a. Look for opportunities to incorporate physical activities into your travel itinerary, such as hiking, swimming, or cycling.

   b. Take advantage of walking or running in new and scenic locations to keep up with your cardio routine.

Portable Equipment and Workout Routines for Workouts on the Go:

1. Resistance Bands:

   a. Discuss the benefits of resistance bands, including their portability, versatility, and ability to provide a full-body workout.

   b. Provide a range of exercises that can be performed with resistance

bands, targeting different muscle groups.
2. Suspension Trainers:
   a. Explain the benefits of suspension trainers for portable workouts, as they can be easily attached to doors or trees.
   b. Demonstrate various exercises that can be done with suspension trainers, focusing on stability and strength training.
3. Jump Rope:
   a. Highlight the advantages of a jump rope, including its compact size and ability to provide an intense cardiovascular workout.
   b. Offer jump rope routines for different fitness levels, incorporating variations such as single jumps, double under, and crisscross.

Utilizing Technology and Online Resources for Home Workouts Away from Home:
1. Fitness Apps and Websites:
   a. List popular fitness apps and websites that offer a wide range of home workout routines and exercise videos.
   b. Discuss the benefits of following guided workout sessions and accessing customized workout plans to suit your fitness goals.
2. Virtual Fitness Communities:
   a. Highlight the importance of connecting with virtual fitness communities when away from home.
   b. Discuss the benefits of joining online fitness groups, participating in challenges, and finding workout buddies for motivation and accountability.
3. Live Streaming Workouts:

a. Inform readers about the availability of live streaming workout sessions, where they can follow along with trainers in real-time.

b. Provide tips on setting up a suitable workout space and ensuring a stable internet connection for uninterrupted sessions.

Traveling does not have to disrupt your fitness routine. By implementing strategies for staying active and maintaining fitness while on the go, utilizing portable equipment and workout routines, and taking advantage of technology and online resources, you can continue your fitness journey regardless of your location.

CHAPTER TEN

Conclusion

Recap of key points covered in the book

Throughout this eBook, we have explored various aspects of building a home gym and crafting an effective workout routine. Let us take a moment to recap some key points that we have covered:

The Importance of a Home Gym: We discussed the convenience and cost-effectiveness of having a home gym. By eliminating the need for a gym membership and providing the freedom to exercise whenever you want, a home gym becomes a valuable asset in achieving your fitness goals.

Setting Up Your Home Gym: We delved into choosing the right equipment based on your fitness goals, available space, and budget. We also provided insights on essential equipment such as cardio machines, strength training tools, and accessories to enhance your workout experience.

Crafting an Effective Workout Routine: We guided you through the process of designing a workout routine tailored to your goals, fitness level, and lifestyle. From warm-up exercises to targeted workouts, we examined the significance of incorporating variety, progression, and recovery into your routine.

Maximizing Results at Home: We explored strategies for achieving optimal results while working out at home. From staying motivated and accountable to incorporating proper nutrition and rest, we highlighted the importance of a holistic approach to fitness.

B. Encouragement for readers to start or enhance their home workout journey

Now that we have covered all the fundamental aspects of fitness at home, I want to reinforce the significance of taking action. It is essential to acknowledge that starting or enhancing your home workout journey may seem intimidating or overwhelming at first. However, I encourage you to embrace the potential that lies within this endeavor. Remember that every fitness journey begins with a single step, and I assure you that taking that first step towards working out at home will be one of the most rewarding decisions you make. The power to transform your body, mind, and overall well-being rests in your hands. Trust in your abilities, stay committed, and watch your resilience grow along with your fitness journey.

Final words of motivation and inspiration for a lifelong commitment to fitness at home.

As we conclude this eBook, I would like to leave you with a final dose of motivation and inspiration. Committing to fitness at home is not just a short-term goal but a lifelong commitment to your health and happiness. By embarking on this journey, you are investing in yourself, your longevity, and your overall quality of life.

Remember that progress is not always linear, and there may be days when you face setbacks or obstacles. During these moments, draw strength from your initial motivation, reminding yourself of why you started in the first place. Embrace the challenges as opportunities for growth and celebrate every small victory along the way.

By prioritizing your well-being and embracing the many benefits of exercising at home, you are not only transforming your body but fostering discipline, self-belief, and resilience.

Stay consistent, seek constant improvement, and cherish the incredible journey that lies ahead. With the knowledge and guidance provided in this eBook, you possess all the tools necessary to succeed on your fitness journey at home. The power to sculpt your dream body, elevate your energy levels, and boost your confidence awaits you. Take the first step today, and unlock your true potential in the comfort of your own home.
Here's to your new chapter of fitness at home. Let this be the beginning of an extraordinary, lifelong commitment to becoming the best version of yourself